EVERYTHING ABOUT

HRM DIET

Complete Nutritional Cookbook, Foods, Meal Plan, Recipes And A Guide To Helping You Lose Weight, Improve Sporting Performance, And Insulin Sensitivity

DR. ALVIN BRANTLEY

Disclaimer

The information provided in this book is intended for general informational purposes only. It is not a substitute for professional medical advice, diagnosis, or treatment.

You should not use the information in this book for diagnosing or treating a health problem or disease by self decision. Always seek the advice of your physician or other qualified health provider with any questions you may have regarding a medical condition.

The author and publisher of this book make no representations or warranties with respect to the accuracy, applicability, fitness, or completeness of the contents of this book. The information contained in this book is based on the author's research and experience, and it is shared with the understanding that the author is not engaged in rendering medical, health, or any other kind of professional advice for you by this book.

The author does not endorse or promote any specific products, brands, or companies related to the contents provided in this book.

Any mention of products or services in this book is for informational purposes only and does not constitute an endorsement.

The author has not entered into any affiliate marketing agreements and has not signed any endorsement deals with individuals, organizations, or companies.

Readers are encouraged to consult with their healthcare providers before making any dietary or lifestyle chaSnges based on the information provided in this book. The author and publisher disclaim any liability for the decisions made by readers based on the information in this book.

ESSENTIALS OF THE HRM DIET

A weight loss strategy based on heart rate management principles is called the HRM (Heart Rate Monitoring) diet. For those looking to lose weight in an efficient and long-lasting way, it is imperative to grasp the fundamentals of heart rate monitoring. Important components of this foundation include the significance of heart rate monitoring, measurement techniques, and goal heart rate zone determination.

CHAPTER ONE

Knowledge Of The HRM Diet

The Heart Rate Monitor Diet, or HRM Diet, is a weight loss strategy that maximizes activity intensity and burns calories by using heart rate monitors. This novel approach adjusts exercise intensity to optimize fat burning and total fitness by accounting for each person's heart rate zones.

The HRM Diet's central tenet is the relationship between heart rate and the body's capacity for effective calorie burning. People can customize their workout regimens to get the best outcomes possible in their weight reduction journey by learning about and adjusting their heart rate zones.

How HRM Can Help You Lose Weight

Heart rate monitor integration with weight reduction plans provides an individualized, data-driven approach to fitness. People can maximize the effectiveness of their workouts by identifying their target heart rate zones by taking accurate heart rate readings while exercising. Consequently, this improves the body's capacity to burn calories, thereby encouraging efficient weight loss. Additionally, HRM offers insightful information about the length and intensity of workouts, assisting people in striking a balance between weight control and cardiovascular health.

Heart Rate Zone Utilization For Best Outcomes

The HRM Diet places a strong emphasis on the value of heart rate zones, each of which denotes a particular workout intensity level.

The resting zone, fat-burning zone, anaerobic zone, aerobic zone, and maximum effort zone are some of these zones. By being aware of and adept at navigating these zones, people can customize their workouts to meet particular objectives. The fat-burning zone is especially important for weight loss since it maximizes the body's usage of fat as its main energy source when exercising.

Personalizing Exercises With HRM

One of the HRM Diet's advantages is its capacity to tailor exercises to each person's fitness level and objectives. People can make sure that their workouts are both difficult and within the ideal heart rate ranges for burning calories by using heart rate monitors. The HRM Diet is a desirable choice for people looking for a more customized and successful approach to fitness because it adds a degree of precision to weight loss attempts.

Heart Rate Monitoring Fundamentals

The knowledge of how heart rate affects the body's reaction to exercise forms the basis of the HRM diet.

Understanding how the heart reacts to exercise and how heart rate affects calorie burn are fundamentals. People can customize their exercise regimens to meet particular weight loss objectives by keeping an eye on their heart rates.

Heart Rate Is Important For Losing Weight

It is impossible to overestimate the importance of heart rate inflation to weight loss. When engaging in physical exercise, a controlled heart rate keeps the body in the ideal fat-burning zone. Based on the science of exercise physiology, this component of the HRM diet emphasizes the relationship between heart rate and the body's capacity to effectively burn calories, which promotes weight loss.

How Your Heart Rate Is Measured

The ability to measure heart rate accurately is essential for putting the HRM diet into practice. Real-time heart rate data can be obtained by techniques including wearable fitness technologies, pulse checks, and heart rate monitors. Accurate measurement enables people to modify the level of intensity during their exercises, making sure they remain in the appropriate heart rate ranges for successful weight reduction.

Zones Of Target Heart Rate

One of the most important parts of the HRM diet is setting target heart rates. These zones are customized for each person depending on specific characteristics including age, degree of fitness, and health. People can maximize their calorie expenditure during exercise and increase the effectiveness of their weight loss attempts by exercising within these preset heart rate levels.

Fundamentals Of The HRM Diet

The HRM diet is based on a set of guidelines that integrate heart rate monitoring with calorie restriction. By maximizing the advantages of both exercise and diet, this dual strategy promotes a weisynergisticallyistic way.

Heart Rate And Calorie Intake

An essential tenet of the HRM diet is the relationship between heart rate and caloric intake.

Keeping track of calories burned and ingested guarantees a proper energy balance that supports weight loss.

A calorie-restricted diet and heart-rate-based exercise regimen help people establish a long-lasting calorie deficit, which is essential for losing extra weight.

Tailoring Diet Programs

The HRM diet acknowledges the value of individualized nutritional strategies. Dietary programs can be customized by adjusting the amount of calories consumed to meet the needs of the individual, accounting for variables like age, gender, degree of exercise, and general health. People can maximize their weight reduction journey and make it long-term maintainable by matching their eating decisions with heart rate-based exercise regimens.

First Things First

A deliberate strategy is needed when starting a weight loss journey, and a key component is creating a Human Resource Management (HRM) diet. This thorough book explores the nuances of integrating dietary methods and HRM for successful weight loss. It's important to comprehend the fundamental steps required in starting this journey of healthy living before getting into the specifics.

Creating an HRM diet plan for weight loss starts with a detailed evaluation of your present fitness level.

This is several number of things, such as your general health, medical background, and physical ability. A pre-workout health check is essential for detecting any possible health issues or restrictions that can affect your capacity to perform specific workouts or make dietary adjustments.

Pre-Workout Medical Exam

Making sure your body is prepared for the demands of a weight reduction program requires you to perform a pre-workout health assessment.

To assess your cardiovascular health, joint integrity, and other critical indications, you should speak with medical professionals.

This is a crucial step in developing a personalized HRM food plan that reduces hazards and fits your specific health demands.

Having Reasonable Objectives

Setting and achieving realistic goals is essential to any weight loss process.

The significance of setting quantifiable goals is discussed in this section, taking into account variables including targeted weight loss, period, and general health gains. Maintaining motivation and a long-term commitment to the HRM diet requires finding a balance between goal and attainability.

CHAPTER TWO

Selecting An Appropriate Heart Rate Monitor

Choosing the right heart rate monitor (HRM) is essential to putting an HRM diet into practice.

This entails comprehending the several kinds of HRMs on the market and assessing their attributes.

An HRM that's well-chosen can help you monitor your heart rate throughout exercise, maximize calorie burn, and make sure that your routines are in line with your weight reduction objectives.

Various Hrm Types

This section explores the many heart rate monitor models that are on the market, from entry-level wearables to high-tech versions. Being able to distinguish between wrist-based monitors, chest strap monitors, and other options will help you make an informed choice depending on your comfort level, preferences, and the particular needs of your HRM diet plan.

Aspects To Take Into Account

It is equally crucial to take into account particular aspects that correspond with your weight loss goals in addition to the different types of HRMs.

This section of the manual examines characteristics including data synchronization capabilities, accuracy, and interoperability with other fitness technologies. By giving careful thought to these aspects, you can make sure that the

HRM you select accurately and insightfully supports your HRM diet and helps you make well-informed decisions.

Creating A Plan For Your Hrm Diet

Starting a weight loss journey necessitates a carefully thought-out plan customized to your particular requirements. For individuals looking for a practical and long-lasting solution, the HRM (High Protein, Moderate Carb) diet is a popular option. You will be guided through the essential steps of developing your own customized HRM food plan by this in-depth guide.

Knowledge Of Macronutrients

Understanding the function of macronutrients in your body is essential to developing a successful HRM diet plan.

The three main macronutrients are proteins, carbohydrates, and lipids. Each has a unique function in promoting general health.

Proteins help build and repair muscles, carbohydrates give us energy, and lipids are necessary for many internal processes. It is essential to consume these macronutrients in a balanced manner if you want to lose weight as effectively as possible.

Carbs, Fats, And Proteins

When it comes to the finer details of each macronutrient, proteins are frequently regarded as the mainstay of an HRM diet. Lean meats, fish, eggs, and legumes are examples of high-protein foods that are essential for maintaining lean muscle mass and boosting satiety during weight loss.

Despite being vilified in some diets, carbohydrates are a necessary source of energy.

A consistent release of energy and the maintenance of stable blood sugar levels is ensured by choosing complex carbs such as whole grains and vegetables.

In the meanwhile, consuming good fats from foods like almonds, avocados, and olive oil promotes general health.

Ensuring Proper Nutrient Ratios

Achieving the proper macronutrient balance is essential to the HRM diet's effectiveness. Finding the ideal balance requires knowledge of your personal requirements, degree of activity, and objectives for weight loss. Although eating more protein is encouraged, it's advisable to consume carbohydrates in moderation. The final piece of the puzzle is balancing good fats, which promotes a nourishing and long-lasting eating strategy.

Creating a Meal Plan

Developing a well-organized meal plan is a cornerstone of the HRM diet. This entails giving careful regard to meal scheduling, portion sizes, and the distribution of macronutrients throughout the day. A well-designed meal plan guarantees that your body gets the nutrients it needs for general health as well as aids in weight loss. Having a nutritionist consult with you can help you create a meal plan that suits your unique requirements and tastes.

Examples of Menus

Sample menus can be a useful tool to offer helpful insights into how the HRM diet should be implemented in practice. These meal plans offer a range of food selections that are in line with the HRM principles and may be used as templates to build your daily or weekly meals. Sample meal plans are flexible and can be customized to meet individual nutritional needs and taste preferences while still following the main guidelines of the HRM diet.

Including HRM Information

Technology has a big impact on fitness and health in the digital era. Adding HRM (Heart Rate Monitor) data to your weight reduction journey gives your plan a more dynamic touch. While exercising, keeping an eye on your heart rate optimizes the burning of calories and guarantees that your workouts are customized to your fitness level. By integrating HRM data, you can take a more customized strategy that will maximize your efforts and improve the overall efficacy of the HRM diet plan.

CHAPTER THREE

Workout And Hrm

Every weight loss program must include exercise, but the HRM diet goes one step further by introducing heart rate monitoring technology. Through comprehension and utilization of your heart rate throughout various forms of physical activity, you may customize your training regimens to optimize fat burning and enhance your general fitness level.

Exercise Is Essential For Losing Weight

It is impossible to overestimate the role exercise plays in weight loss. Frequent exercise increases metabolism, strengthens the heart, and improves muscle tone in addition to burning calories. Recognizing the importance of exercise in attaining long-term, sustainable weight loss, the HRM diet places a high focus on it.

Exercise For The Heart

Running, cycling, and swimming are examples of cardiovascular exercises that are essential to an HRM diet. By increasing heart rate, these exercises encourage burning calories and reducing body fat. During aerobic exercises, the HRM helps you stay in the ideal fat-burning zone by giving you real-time data on your heart rate.

Strength Development

Another important component of the HRM diet is adding strength training to your exercise regimen. Strength training increases lean muscle mass, which in turn improves the body's capacity to burn calories at rest, whereas cardio burns calories throughout the workout.

The HRM assists in monitoring the degree of intensity during strength training, ensuring that you reach the ideal point for the best outcomes.

Optimizing Exercise Using HRM

Your workouts will be more effective if you use the HRM as a useful tool. You can adjust the length and intensity of your exercise sessions to meet your weight loss objectives by keeping an eye on your heart rate. This tailored approach increases the effectiveness of your workouts by making them more focused and goal-oriented.

Keep An Eye On Intensity

Monitoring exercise intensity is one of the main advantages of using an HRM in your fitness regimen.

By giving you access to real-time heart rate data, the gadget assists you in maintaining optimal fat burning within designated heart rate ranges. This degree of accuracy guarantees that you are exercising and doing so at a level that encourages weight loss.

Tailoring Exercises

The HRM diet promotes tailoring exercise regimens to each person's fitness objectives and level of fitness.

A person's exercise regimen can be customized to meet their demands by knowing how different heart rate zones affect calorie burn.

By ensuring that workouts are both pleasurable and effective, this customization helps to increase adherence to the overall weight loss strategy.

The HRM diet uses heart rate monitoring to increase the efficiency of exercise, bringing technology into the weight loss process.

This strategy, which acknowledges the value of both strength and cardio training, enables customized and targeted workouts, which eventually contribute to a more effective and long-lasting weight loss journey.

Observing Development

Efficient management of weight reduction frequently entails the careful monitoring of multiple factors to assess advancement.

The Heart Rate Monitor is a useful tool in this quest (HRM). Making educated changes to food and exercise is made possible by having a thorough grasp of the body's reaction through the use of HRM data for progress tracking.

CHAPTER FOUR

Using HRM Information To Monitor Progress

Heart rate monitors provide real-time information on how hard a person is working out and how much effort they are putting in. People can keep an extensive record of their workouts by synchronizing HRM data with fitness apps or gadgets. This information becomes an invaluable tool for comprehending the relationship between heart rate, caloric expenditure, and the efficacy of various exercise regimens.

Examining Trends In Heart Rate

When heart rate trends are analyzed over time, patterns emerge that may indicate how the body has adjusted to activity. Consistent drops in resting heart rate could indicate enhanced cardiovascular health, but variations during exercise can identify the ideal levels of intensity. Comprehending these patterns enables individuals to customize their workout regimens for optimal efficacy and efficiency.

Modifying Exercise And Diet

There is more to using HRM data in the weight reduction process than just monitoring calories burned. It acts as a guide for modifying exercise and food to meet personal objectives. For example, knowing which heart rate ranges maximize fat burning can help with cardio exercises, and keeping track of calories burned can help with developing a diet that is balanced and promotes weight loss.

Extra Tools For Monitoring

Although HRMs provide insightful information, using other monitoring instruments improves the tracking procedure as a whole. Technology that gauges stress levels, quality of sleep, and general well-being offers a more comprehensive picture of the variables affecting weight reduction. This all-encompassing strategy enables focused treatments to address certain issues.

Weight Monitoring

Even with heart rate monitoring's subtleties, conventional measurements like weight tracking are still crucial for assessing overall development. When combined with frequent weigh-ins, HRM data provides a more thorough picture of the weight loss process. It gives people a comprehensive understanding of their efforts by enabling them to connect variations in body weight with changes in heart rate patterns.

Body Dimensions

Monitoring body measures is essential for recording changes in body composition in addition to weight. While HRM data can indicate gains in cardiovascular health and fitness, measures of the waist, hips, and other important body parts offer a more concrete picture of changes in muscle mass and body fat. Setting reasonable and attainable goals is made easier with this all-encompassing approach, which guarantees a more nuanced knowledge of success.

a multimodal approach to progress tracking is made possible by the incorporation of HRM data into weight loss management. People can make decisions that are in line with their own goals by doing everything from evaluating heart rate patterns to modifying their diet and exercise routine. To obtain a thorough picture of an individual's weight loss journey, it is recommended to complement HRM insights with conventional metrics like body measurements and weight tracking.

CHAPTER FIVE

Fixing Issues And Faqs

People who start the HRM Diet may encounter several difficulties and unknowns. This section explores typical troubleshooting situations and commonly asked issues, offering advice and methods to get beyond any obstacles.

Typical Obstacles In HRM Dieting

Even while the HRM Diet has some potential benefits, there may be some difficulties along the way. Common problems include weight reduction plateaus, trouble adjusting to HRM monitoring, and misgivings regarding the accuracy of HRMs. This section tackles these issues and provides solutions to keep up the momentum towards your weight loss objectives.

Standstill

Concerns about weight reduction plateaus are prevalent among people following any diet, including the HRM Diet. Sustained growth depends on comprehending the causes of plateaus and putting effective tactics in place to overcome them. This section examines the causes of plateaus and offers tweaks to jump-start weight reduction.

Getting Used To Monitoring HRM

Making the switch to HRM monitoring can be difficult, particularly for people who are not familiar with the technique. This part offers tips on adjusting to HRM use, comprehending the data it produces, and making the most of its advantages for diet and workout regimen optimization.

Answers To Common Questions

This section answers several commonly asked questions about the HRM Diet. People can discover thorough answers to improve their comprehension and adherence to the HRM Diet, answering anything from questions concerning the accuracy of HRMs to uncertainties regarding the synergy between diet and exercise.

HRM Precision

A crucial component of the HRM Diet's effectiveness is accurate monitoring. This section examines the accuracy of HRMs and addresses myths and worries about how accurate they are at monitoring heart rate and energy expenditure. By making these points clear, people may be sure they can rely on the information their HRMs give to make well-informed decisions.

Exercise And Diet Questions

One essential element of the HRM Diet is combining exercise and nutrition. However, questions can surface regarding how well these two components work together.

This section answers frequently asked questions and offers information on how, within the parameters of the HRM Diet, diet and activity complement one another to maximize weight reduction outcomes.

CHAPTER SIX

Upholding AN HEALTHY STYLE

Maintaining a healthy lifestyle is an essential component of successful weight management. This includes a comprehensive strategy that emphasizes long-term habits rather than fad diets. Sustainable routines, frequent physical activity, and a balanced diet are the cornerstones of a healthy lifestyle that promotes weight loss.

Long-Term Plans For Maintaining Your Weight

The goal of weight management is to maintain a healthy weight over the long run, not only to drop pounds. Setting reasonable and doable objectives, including a range of nutrient-dense foods in one's diet, and adopting a lifestyle that promotes general well-being are all long-term tactics for maintaining a healthy weight. Rather than focusing on band-aid solutions, these tactics emphasize small, long-term improvements.

Healthy Eating Practices

An important factor in reaching and keeping a healthy weight is developing sustainable eating habits. This entails selecting foods carefully, as well as how often and in what portions to eat. Lean proteins, whole grains, healthy fats, and a range of fruits and vegetables all contribute to a balanced diet that promotes metabolism, keeps energy levels stable, and helps ward off nutritional deficiencies. Sustainable eating practices also include exercising moderation and being conscious of emotional or mindless eating.

Regular Exercise Schedules

Frequent exercise is essential to any effective weight-loss strategy. Regular exercise regimens improve general health and well-being in addition to calorie expenditure. Including aerobic, strength, and flexibility activities in a routine promotes fat burning, the development of lean muscle mass, and enhanced metabolic function. Exercise can become a sustainable component of a healthy lifestyle by selecting interesting things to engage in. Consistency is the key to this.

Maintaining a healthy lifestyle, using long-term weight maintenance techniques, developing sustainable food habits, and participating in regular exercise routines are all components of a holistic approach to weight control.

People can accomplish their weight loss objectives and maintain a healthy weight over time by addressing these factors collectively.

It's critical to see weight control as a lifelong process that embraces small, sustainable adjustments that improve well-being in general.

The HRM Diet's emphasis on customization is one of its main advantages. Given that people have different tastes and difficulties, this diet promotes adjusting the strategy to meet individual requirements. Customization lies at the core of the HRM Diet, whether it is adding fun activities, deciding on favorite meals within a given calorie limit, or picking particular workout routines.

Putting Motivational Strategies Into Practice:

Successful weight loss depends on motivation, and the HRM Diet uses techniques for motivation that are frequently used in HRM. This entails establishing SMART objectives (Specific,

Measurable, Achievable, Relevant, Time-Bound), giving encouragement, and cultivating a sense of success. When weight loss goals are in line with personal goals, people are more likely to maintain motivation as they progress.

Establishing Accountability Frameworks:

Accountability is essential to the HRM Diet because it drives success. Expanding upon the notion of performance management, people are urged to set up accountability frameworks, such as attending support groups, keeping a food diary, or working out with a spouse. These methods foster a sense of accountability for one's health in addition to improving diet compliance.

Observation And Reaction:

The HRM Diet takes its cues from human resource management performance appraisal systems, with regular monitoring and feedback being key components.

People can make well-informed modifications to their weight loss plan by monitoring their success. This entails evaluating both achievements and failures to make necessary adjustments and allow for ongoing improvement.

Tracking Development And Modifying Objectives

People can accurately measure their progress and make necessary adjustments to their weight loss objectives by regularly monitoring their heart rate data. Through the analysis of heart rate changes during exercise, people can pinpoint areas in which they are either plateauing or need improvement. The HRM Diet's flexibility is one of its main advantages since it enables a dynamic and flexible approach to weight loss, ensuring that participants stay on track and keep making progress toward their objectives.

HRM And Nutrition Together

To successfully lose weight, nutrition is just as important as exercise when following the HRM Diet. Overall results are improved when the HRM technique is used with a healthy, balanced diet. People may enhance their recuperation, sustain their energy levels, and maximize the efficiency of their exercise regimens by providing their bodies with the proper nutrition. Within the parameters of the HRM Diet, targeted activity and healthy eating combine to provide a comprehensive approach to weight loss.

Overcoming Obstacles And Maintaining Motivation

The HRM Diet has drawbacks, just like any other weight-loss plan. It takes perseverance, commitment, and a desire to comprehend and address each person's unique physiological reactions. It's important to maintain motivation along the way, and the HRM Diet promotes setting reasonable objectives, acknowledging minor accomplishments, and keeping an eye on the long-term advantages of better health and fitness.

Conclusion

In conclusion, by incorporating human resource management concepts, the HRM Diet presents a fresh and successful strategy for weight loss. Customization, accountability frameworks, motivational techniques, and ongoing monitoring enable people to design long-term plans that suit their tastes and objectives. It is crucial to stress the value of encouragement for ongoing success as we consider the major ideas covered in this nutritional strategy.

This examination of the HRM Diet has brought attention to several important ideas. These include the necessity of ongoing monitoring and feedback, the personalization of weight loss plans, the incorporation of motivational tactics, and the creation of accountability mechanisms. By understanding these ideas, people can use the HRM Diet to help them lose weight and motivate them to stick to a long-term healthy lifestyle.

Motivation For Ongoing Achievement:

It's admirable to start a weight loss journey, and the HRM Diet offers a structure that extends beyond food limitations. Encouraging people to succeed in the future is essential as they overcome obstacles and recognize their accomplishments. Sustaining motivation is essential to making the HRM Diet a lifelong tool for maintaining a healthy weight and general well-being, whether through self-reflection, outside support networks, or acknowledging accomplishments.

9 798869 594723